# FINDING ZEN

## A Beginner's Guide to Yoga

### Philipp Frühwirth

# CONTENTS

# INTRODUCTION TO YOGA: A COMPLETE GUIDE FOR BEGINNERS

Yoga is an ancient practice that originated in India over 5,000 years ago. It involves a combination of physical postures, breathing techniques, meditation, and relaxation exercises. Yoga has been known to provide numerous health benefits to individuals who practice it regularly, including stress reduction, increased flexibility and strength, improved cardiovascular health, and enhanced mental clarity.

If you are new to yoga, it can seem overwhelming and daunting. However, by following the right advice and tips, you can start your yoga journey with confidence and ease. This guide is designed to provide a comprehensive overview of yoga and help you get started on the path to greater health and well-being.

**Yoga Basics**

Yoga is an exercise that can be practiced by people of all fitness levels and ages. In order to practice yoga, you will need to get comfortable with some basic terminology.

Asana - the physical postures or poses used in yoga
Pranayama - the breathing techniques used in yoga
Mantra - a phrase or word that is repeated during meditation
Mudra - hand gestures used to focus energy during meditation
Chakra - energy centers in the body
Om - a mantra that is often chanted in yoga practice

**Equipment**

One of the best things about yoga is that you don't need a lot of equipment to get started. All you really need is a yoga mat and comfortable clothing.

The right yoga mat will provide you with the necessary cushioning and grip to help you perform the yoga poses safely and effectively. Choose a mat that is thick and has a non-slip surface to prevent slips and falls.

Clothing should be comfortable and allow for freedom of movement. Look for breathable fabrics that allow your skin to breathe, such as cotton, linen, or bamboo.

**Types of Yoga**

There are many different types of yoga, each with its own focus and benefits. Some popular types of yoga include:

Hatha Yoga - focuses on physical postures and breathing techniques
Vinyasa Yoga - a dynamic form of yoga that flows from pose to pose
Restorative Yoga - uses props to support the body in poses for extended periods
Ashtanga Yoga - a fast-paced, physically demanding form of yoga
Bikram Yoga - a specific form of hot yoga that involves a sequence of 26 poses performed in a heated room

Conclusion

Yoga is a holistic practice that provides numerous physical and mental health benefits. If you are new to yoga, start with the basics and choose a style that suits your needs and preferences. With regular practice, you will experience increased flexibility, strength, and endurance, and create a greater sense of peace and inner calm.

# UNDERSTANDING THE BENEFITS OF YOGA FOR YOUR MIND AND BODY

Yoga is a holistic approach to physical and mental health that originated in ancient India. Today, it has become increasingly popular worldwide, as people have acknowledged its numerous benefits for the mind and body. The practice of yoga involves a combination of physical asanas (postures), pranayama (breathing), and meditation. When practiced regularly, it can bring about profound positive changes in your physical, emotional, and spiritual health.

One of the main benefits of yoga is its ability to reduce stress and anxiety. Studies have shown that yoga and meditation practices can help reduce cortisol, a hormone produced in response to stress. This, in turn, can help improve mood, reduce symptoms of anxiety and depression, and increase the ability to cope with daily stressors.

The physical asanas of yoga also offer many benefits to the body. Regular practice can help increase flexibility, strength, balance, and stability. It can also help reduce the risk of injuries, as well as manage chronic pain conditions such as arthritis and back pain. Yoga is also an ideal form of low-impact exercise for people of all ages, including seniors.

In addition to physical benefits, yoga can also lead to profound changes in the practitioner's spiritual and emotional health. Yoga encourages self-awareness and introspection, helping individuals to become more mindful of their thoughts, emotions, and actions. This can lead to improved emotional regulation, increased self-esteem, and greater self-acceptance.

Another significant benefit of yoga is its ability to promote a deep sense of relaxation and inner peace. The combination of physical postures, breathing techniques, and meditation can help reduce to release tension and promote a state of deep relaxation, allowing practitioners to experience a greater sense of calm and inner peace.

In conclusion, the practice of yoga offers numerous benefits for both the mind and body. By reducing stress and anxiety, improving physical fitness, and promoting mental clarity and relaxation, yoga has become a popular form of exercise and self-care for people of all ages and backgrounds. Whether you're new to yoga or an experienced practitioner, incorporating this ancient practice into your daily routine can bring about profound positive changes in your mental, physical, and spiritual health.

# THE DIFFERENT STYLES OF YOGA AND WHAT THEY CAN OFFER

Yoga is a practice that has been around for centuries and has evolved into various styles. The word "yoga" itself derives from the Sanskrit word "yuj," which means "to yoke" or "to unite." The primary objective of all yoga styles is to unite the mind, body, and spirit. Different styles of yoga have been developed to cater to different needs, body types, and lifestyles.

**Here are some of the most popular styles of yoga and what they can offer:**

1. Hatha Yoga: Hatha yoga is the most common and fundamental form of yoga. It focuses on basic postures or "asanas," breathing techniques, and relaxation. This style is perfect for beginners as it allows them to learn the fundamentals of yoga.

2. Vinyasa Yoga: Vinyasa yoga is a more fluid and dynamic style that synchronizes movement with breath. It is a fast-paced style that is popular with those who want to sweat and strengthen their muscles.

3. Ashtanga Yoga: Ashtanga yoga follows a set series of postures that are performed in a specific order. It is physically demanding and involves six series of specific postures, so it is ideal for those who want a more structured yoga practice.

4. Iyengar Yoga: Iyengar yoga is a meticulous and focused style that emphasizes proper alignment to prevent injuries. Props such as straps, blocks, and blankets are often used to help practitioners get into the correct postures.

5. Bikram Yoga: Bikram yoga, also known as hot yoga, is a style that is practiced in a heated room. The temperature is typically set to 105 degrees Fahrenheit with 40% humidity. This style aims to boost flexibility and help with detoxification.

6. Yin Yoga: Yin yoga is a slow-paced style that involves holding postures for longer periods. This style targets the connective tissues such as ligaments, tendons, and fascia, promoting flexibility.

7. Restorative Yoga: Restorative yoga is a calming and gentle style that involves holding postures for several minutes with the use of props such as bolsters, blankets, and blocks. This style aims to promote relaxation and stress reduction.

Each style of yoga offers unique benefits, and it's essential to find a style that suits your needs and goals. It's worth trying different styles to find the one that resonates with you and where you feel comfortable. Remember, there are no rules or expectations in yoga practice, and it's ultimately about finding a practice that nourishes your body, mind, and soul.

# BEST YOGA POSES FOR FLEXIBILITY AND STRENGTH

Yoga has emerged as one of the best forms of exercise for overall fitness and health. It combines physical and mental exercises that help to improve flexibility, strength, balance, and mental clarity. Practicing yoga can help you increase your flexibility, tone and strengthen muscles and boost your metabolism.

**Here are some of the best yoga poses for improving flexibility and strength:**

1. Downward Dog Pose (Adho Mukha Svanasana): This pose helps increase strength in your arms and shoulder, lengthen your spine and hamstrings, and release any tension in your lower back.

2. Warrior Pose (Virabhadrasana): This pose strengthens your legs, improves balance, and open your hips and chest.

3. Tree Pose (Vrksasana): This pose requires balance and helps to strengthen the muscles in your legs, tones the abdominal muscles and improves concentration.

4. Bound Angle Pose (Baddha Konasana): This pose stretches the inner thighs and groin area, improves flexibility in the knees and hips, and helps to reduce stress.

5. Triangle Pose (Trikonasana): This pose strengthens the lower body, stretches the hamstrings and hips, and increases mobility in the spine.

6. Chair Pose (Utkatasana): This pose strengthens your legs, opens your chest, and tones the abdominal muscles.

7. Boat Pose (Navasana): This pose strengthens your core muscles,

including your abdominal muscles, while also improving balance and concentration.

8. Cobra Pose (Bhujangasana): This pose strengthens the back muscles, hips, and shoulders, while also increasing flexibility in the spine.

9. Half Moon Pose (Ardha Chandrasana): This pose strengthens the legs and core, while also improving balance, stability, and flexibility.

10. Camel Pose (Ustrasana): This pose strengthens the muscles of the back, opens up the chest and throat, and stretches the hips.

These are just a few of the many yoga poses that can help you improve your flexibility and strength. Practicing yoga regularly can benefit your physical and mental health, and these poses are a great place to start. Remember to always listen to your body and work at your own pace. Over time, you will notice significant improvements in your flexibility, strength and overall well-being.

# HOW TO DEVELOP A DAILY YOGA ROUTINE THAT WORKS FOR YOU

Yoga has numerous benefits for the mind and body, and one of the best ways to experience these benefits is through a daily yoga practice. However, developing a daily yoga routine can be challenging, especially if you're unsure where to begin or how to make it work with your busy schedule. Here are some tips for creating a daily yoga practice that works for you.

1. Make it manageable: Start small and build gradually. Even just 10 minutes of yoga a day can be beneficial. As you become more comfortable with the routine, you can slowly increase the duration of your practice.

2. Choose a time that works for you: Decide on a time of day that works with your schedule and lifestyle. Some people prefer to practice in the morning to start their day off right, while others prefer to practice in the evening to wind down after a long day.

3. Find a quiet space: Choose a quiet and peaceful space in your home where you feel comfortable practicing yoga. Ensure that the space has enough room for your mat and any props you may need.

4. Plan your practice: Plan your yoga practice ahead of time so you have a set routine to follow. This will help you stay committed to your daily practice and ensure that you're getting the most out of it.

5. Use online resources: There are many online resources available for creating a daily yoga practice. Consider signing up for online yoga classes or using yoga apps that offer pre-set routines or

customized plans.

6. Listen to your body: Pay attention to your body when practicing yoga. If something doesn't feel right, modify or skip the pose. It's important to honor your body and give it what it needs to avoid injury and maintain a sustainable practice.

7. Make it fun: Incorporate different styles of yoga, poses, and music into your practice to keep things interesting and enjoyable. Remember, yoga is meant to be a practice of self-love and self-care, so make it something that you look forward to each day.

In conclusion, developing a daily yoga routine is a great way to improve your overall health and well-being. By following these tips, you can create a practice that fits your unique needs and lifestyle, helping you reap the many benefits of yoga.

# YOGA FOR WEIGHT LOSS: HOW IT HELPS TO SHED THOSE EXTRA POUNDS

Yoga can provide a complete workout that targets not only the body but also the mind, leading to overall fitness and a sense of well-being. This mind-body discipline originated in India and has been practiced for thousands of years.

While many people associate yoga with relaxation and meditation, it can also be an effective tool for weight loss. Yoga utilizes physical postures (asanas), breathing techniques (pranayama), and meditation to strengthen and tone muscles, increase flexibility, and reduce stress.

Yoga can help you lose weight by increasing your metabolism, which is the rate at which your body burns calories. Certain yoga poses can also help reduce body fat by targeting specific areas of the body. For instance, the sun salutation sequence, consisting of 12 different poses, is an effective way to burn calories and tone muscles in the arms, legs, and abs.

Power yoga and hot yoga are particularly effective for weight loss. Power yoga is a vigorous and fast-paced form of yoga that incorporates dynamic movements and challenging poses to tone muscles and burn calories. Hot yoga, also known as Bikram yoga, is performed in a heated room, and the elevated temperature can help you sweat out toxins and burn more calories.

In addition to the physical benefits, yoga can also help promote healthy eating habits and reduce stress-related eating. Many people turn to food as a way to cope with stress, anxiety, and other negative emotions. Yoga can help you develop mindfulness and self-awareness, which can help you identify and manage stress in a healthier way.

If you are new to yoga, it is recommended to start with a beginner's class and work your way up gradually. As with any exercise program, it is important to consult with your healthcare provider before starting a new practice, especially if you have any health conditions.

In conclusion, yoga is an effective and natural way to lose weight and improve overall health and well-being. By incorporating yoga into your daily routine, you can achieve physical fitness, mental clarity, and inner peace.

# THE ART OF MEDITATION AND YOGA: STRENGTHENING YOUR MIND-BODY CONNECTION

Meditation and yoga are two powerful practices that have been around for thousands of years. They are often practiced together and are known to help strengthen the mind-body connection. Meditation involves training the mind to focus on a single object or thought, while yoga is a combination of physical poses, breathing techniques, and meditation.

Through the practice of meditation and yoga, individuals can achieve a state of calmness and relaxation. This calm state of mind can help manage stress and anxiety, improve focus and concentration, and even reduce symptoms of depression.

Yoga and meditation encourage mindfulness, which means being fully present in the current moment. This practice requires paying attention to physical sensations and breathing patterns, helping to create a sense of inner peace and calm. As the mind and body become more connected, individuals can become more aware of their thoughts, feelings, and bodily sensations, allowing them to manage these more effectively.

Yoga and meditation have been shown to lower cortisol levels, which is the hormone released in response to stress. By reducing cortisol levels, individuals can experience a range of health benefits, such as improved immune function, lower blood pressure, and reduced inflammation.

In addition to stress management, yoga and meditation can also improve flexibility, balance, and range of motion. Yoga poses are designed to stretch and strengthen muscles, while also improving balance and coordination. Breathing techniques used in yoga can also help regulate the nervous system, leading to a calmer state of mind and improved physical health.

The combination of yoga and meditation can enhance the mind-body connection, leading to a greater sense of well-being. Integrating these practices into daily life can help reduce stress, improve mental clarity, and promote physical health. Whether practiced together or separately, meditation and yoga can be an effective tool for achieving a greater sense of inner peace and happiness.

# FINDING INNER PEACE THROUGH YOGA: MEDITATION AND RELAXATION TECHNIQUES

Yoga has long been known as an excellent way to improve physical health, but what many people don't realize is that it can also help to calm and focus the mind. The union of the mind, body, and breath is where the real magic of yoga lies, and mastering this union can help you achieve inner peace and tranquility. In this chapter, we'll explore the art of meditation and some relaxation techniques that can help you deepen your yoga practice and find that inner peace.

Meditation is a powerful tool for calming the mind and reducing stress. By sitting quietly and focusing on your breath or a specific mantra, you can cultivate a sense of inner peace and relaxation. There are many different types of meditation, but one of the most common in yoga is mindfulness meditation. This involves focusing on the present moment and observing your thoughts without judgment. By bringing your attention to the present moment and letting go of distractions, you can release mental tension and anxiety.

Another technique that can be very effective for relaxation is deep breathing, or pranayama. Deep breathing involves slow, full inhales and exhales, which can help to calm the nervous system and reduce stress. One common breathing exercise in yoga is called Nadi Shodhana, or alternate nostril breathing. This involves closing off one nostril at a time and breathing in and out through each nostril in turn. This technique can help to balance the left and right sides of the brain and promote relaxation.

In addition to meditation and breathing techniques, there are many yoga poses that can help to calm the mind and reduce stress. One of the simplest is Savasana, or corpse pose. This involves lying flat on your back with your arms and legs relaxed and your eyes closed. Savasana is often used as a relaxation pose at the end of a yoga practice, but it can also be done on its own as a way to reduce stress and tension.

Other yoga poses that can be effective for relaxation include forward bends, such as Uttanasana (standing forward bend) and Paschimottanasana (seated forward bend). These poses help to calm the mind and release tension in the neck, shoulders, and back. Inversions, such as Salamba Sirsasana (supported headstand) and Viparita Karani (legs up the wall pose), can also be effective for relaxation, as they help to calm the nervous system and promote peacefulness.

In conclusion, yoga is not just a physical practice – it can also be a powerful tool for cultivating inner peace and tranquility. By combining meditation, breathing techniques, and yoga poses, you can deepen your practice and find greater relaxation and calm both on and off the mat. Try incorporating these techniques into your daily routine and see how they can help you find greater balance and peace in your life.

# YOGA BREATHING TECHNIQUES TO REDUCE STRESS AND ANXIETY

Yoga is a great way to relax and reduce stress levels, and breathing techniques play a vital role in achieving this. According to yoga philosophy, pranayama or controlled breathing is believed to be a powerful tool for balancing the emotions and calming the mind. By practicing yoga breathing techniques, one can learn to control the breath and bring awareness to the present moment, creating a sense of relaxation and inner peace.

**Here are some of the best yoga breathing techniques that can help reduce stress and anxiety:**

1. Diaphragmatic breathing: Also known as belly breathing, this technique involves breathing deeply into the belly, filling up the lungs, and releasing the breath slowly. This technique is helpful in reducing the physical symptoms of anxiety such as muscle tension and shortness of breath.

2. Alternate nostril breathing: This technique involves inhaling and exhaling through alternate nostrils while holding one nostril closed with the thumb. This practice is said to help balance the mind, calm the nervous system, and increase mental clarity.

3. Ujjayi breathing: Also known as ocean breath or victorious breath, this technique involves breathing in and out through the nose while constricting the back of the throat, creating a soft hissing sound. This practice can help calm the mind and reduce stress levels.

4. Bhramari breathing: This technique involves inhaling deeply

and then exhaling while making a humming sound like a bee. This practice is highly useful in reducing stress and anxiety levels and promoting relaxation.

5. Kapalabhati breathing: This technique involves rapid and forceful exhalations from the belly while inhaling passively through the nose. This practice helps to clear the mind, energize the body, and reduce feelings of stress and anxiety.

It is important to remember that yoga breathing techniques are not a cure for anxiety, but they can be a useful tool to manage symptoms. Practicing these techniques can help to calm the body and mind, enabling you to feel more balanced, centered, and at peace. With regular practice, yoga breathing techniques can become a valuable part of your self-care routine.

# ADVANCED YOGA POSES FOR THE EXPERIENCED YOGI: CHALLENGING YOUR BODY AND MIND

Yoga, as a practice, is a blend of stretches, movements, and breathing exercises that help you concentrate while challenging your body physically. For beginners, asanas or poses like the downward-facing dog or the corpse pose can be an excellent starting point. On the other hand, advanced students can try moves like the crow pose, scorpion, or the dancer pose.

**Here are some advanced yoga poses that will help experienced and advanced yogis challenge themselves:**

1. Natarajasana (Dancer Pose): This pose is excellent for opening up the heart chakra while also providing a good stretch for the quads and ankles. The dancer pose is not easy to master as it requires balance, strength, and coordination. It involves stretching the arm and leg on the same side while keeping the other arm and leg up in the air.

2. Eka Pada Koundinyasana II (Flying Splits Pose): This pose involves arm balancing and building strength in your core, arms, and hips. It entails entering into an arm balance pose while your leg extends behind you in the air.

3. Handstand Scorpion (Vrischikasana): Merging the strength of the triceps and core, the scorpion pose can be challenging for even the most experienced yogis. It requires a handstand position while simultaneously lifting the legs above the head and placing the feet on the back to form an arch.

4. Firefly Pose (Tittibhasana): This yoga posture concentrates on developing your balancing act, lower belly, and flexibility. It requires spreading the legs widely and placing your hands between them while leaning forward and doing a palm-rest.

5. Peacock Pose (Mayurasana): This pose strengthens the forearms, back, and abdominal muscles. It involves lifting feet and pressing them against the ground while keeping the weight on the arms and elbows.

When practicing advanced yoga poses, it's essential to remember that every body is unique, and so is their journey. Proceeding in a gradual manner while paying attention to one's body is recommended. Pushing beyond the point of discomfort and pain might do more harm than good. It's always advisable to seek professional help from a trained yoga teacher if there's any doubt or discomfort during yoga practice, especially with advanced poses.

In conclusion, advanced yoga poses are for experienced yogis looking to challenge their practice as they take their physical and mental understanding of yoga to the next level. Our bodies are all different, and so each pose is unique to the individual, but adding more challenging postures to our practice will undoubtedly help to strengthen our physical and mental consciousness.

# YOGA THERAPY: HEALING YOUR BODY AND MIND THROUGH YOGA

Yoga therapy is an innovative way to heal and improve mental and physical health. Yoga therapy is based on the ancient science of yoga that helps promote healing and well-being. It focuses on the use of yoga postures, pranayama (breathing), meditation, and other yoga-based techniques to treat specific mental and physical health conditions.

Yoga therapy can be used to treat a wide range of mental and physical health conditions like depression, anxiety, chronic pain, and addiction. The practice of yoga therapy involves working with a trained yoga therapist who is skilled in assessing and identifying specific health problems and devising individualized yoga therapy plans to achieve optimal results.

The therapeutic application of yoga has been found to be particularly effective in treating both acute and chronic physical pain. Chronic pain is a common health concern that affects millions of people and can lead to depression and anxiety. Yoga therapy has been found to be particularly helpful in reducing pain levels, increasing flexibility, and improving overall functioning.

Yoga therapy can also be used to treat mental health conditions such as depression and anxiety. The deep breathing and relaxation techniques used in yoga help to reduce stress, which in turn can help relieve depression and anxiety. Yoga has been found to be particularly effective for individuals suffering from post-traumatic stress disorder (PTSD), as it helps relieve symptoms such as anxiety, flashbacks, and nightmares.

Apart from being a complementary therapy to traditional medicine, yoga therapy can also be used as a standalone treatment for various mental and physical ailments. It has been found to be particularly effective in treating addiction and substance abuse disorders. Yoga therapy can help individuals recover from addiction by providing them with tools to help with stress management, relaxation, and emotional regulation.

In conclusion, yoga therapy is a safe and effective way to treat various physical and mental health conditions. Individuals who are interested in exploring yoga therapy should work with a trained yoga therapist who can develop an individualized treatment plan that addresses their unique needs and goals. With regular practice, yoga therapy has the potential to improve overall health and well-being, both physically and mentally.

# YOGA AND AGING: STAYING ACTIVE AND HEALTHY AS YOU GET OLDER

## Introduction:

Yoga is a holistic discipline that aims to cultivate good health and wellbeing by integrating the mind, body, and spirit. As we age, our bodies and minds undergo significant changes that can lead to a variety of health issues, including joint pain, stiffness, balance problems, and cognitive decline. Fortunately, yoga offers a safe and effective way to stay active and healthy as we get older. This chapter will explore how yoga can improve the physical, mental, and emotional wellbeing of seniors.

## Physical Benefits:

One of the most obvious benefits of yoga for seniors is improved flexibility, balance, and strength. In fact, research shows that regular yoga practice can help to increase bone density, reduce joint pain, and prevent falls. Moreover, the physical postures or asanas of yoga help to promote circulation, boost the immune system, and reduce inflammation, which can have a positive impact on overall health and longevity.

## Mental Benefits:

Yoga is also renowned for its mental health benefits, including stress reduction, anxiety relief, and improved sleep quality. As we age, we may become more prone to stress, depression, and anxiety due to changes in our lifestyle or health. Yoga can help to calm the mind, promote a sense of relaxation, and enhance mental clarity and focus.

**Emotional Benefits:**

Finally, yoga can have a significant impact on emotional wellbeing. By practicing mindfulness and self-awareness, yoga helps to cultivate greater self-acceptance, compassion, and resilience. This, in turn, can lead to a greater sense of happiness, peace, and contentment.

Conclusion:

In conclusion, yoga is an excellent practice for seniors who wish to stay active, healthy, and mentally sharp. By incorporating a regular yoga practice into your lifestyle, you can reap numerous benefits that promote overall wellbeing, including improved physical fitness, reduced stress and anxiety, and greater emotional resilience.

# THE POWER OF YOGA IN CHRONIC PAIN MANAGEMENT

Chronic pain is a common condition that affects millions of people worldwide. It can be caused by a variety of physical and mental health problems, including injuries, arthritis, fibromyalgia, and depression. For many individuals, chronic pain can disrupt daily life, making it difficult to work, exercise, and even socialize. Pain medications may offer temporary relief, but they often come with side effects that can be unpleasant and even harmful.

Yoga has been shown to be a useful complementary therapy for individuals with chronic pain. It offers a natural, non-invasive way to manage symptoms and improve daily function. The practice of yoga involves physical postures, breathing exercises, and meditation techniques that work together to enhance mind-body awareness and relaxation. Here are some ways in which yoga can help individuals with chronic pain:

1. Increases Joint Flexibility and Mobility

Yoga postures, or asanas, can help to stretch and strengthen the muscles and joints, improving flexibility and mobility. This can be especially beneficial for those with chronic pain caused by conditions such as arthritis, as it helps to reduce stiffness and inflammation.

2. Enhances Relaxation

Yoga involves deep breathing techniques and meditation, which have been shown to reduce stress and tension in the body. By calming the mind and body, a person may experience a decrease in pain due to the release of endorphins, which are natural painkillers.

## 3. Builds Strength and Endurance

Many yoga poses require strength and endurance to hold, with modifications available for different levels of learners. Regular yoga practice can help individuals build up strength and stamina, which may help to reduce chronic pain symptoms.

## 4. Improves Sleep Quality

Chronic pain can disrupt sleep, leading to fatigue and even worse chronic pain. Studies have found that regular yoga practice can improve sleep quality, helping individuals with chronic pain to feel more rested and energized.

## 5. Enhances Mind-Body Connection

Yoga involves the mind-body connection, which can be beneficial for individuals with chronic pain due to its potential to enhance body awareness and control. By practicing mindfulness and meditation techniques, individuals may develop a greater capacity to focus on and regulate their pain experience.

Yoga offers many benefits to individuals with chronic pain, reducing the need for medications and other invasive treatments. However, it is important to consult with a healthcare professional before beginning a yoga practice, especially if chronic pain is affecting your functional capacities. A qualified yoga teacher can create a modified practice appropriate to your pain level, physical fitness, and overall health needs.

# YOGA FOR ATHLETES: ENHANCING FLEXIBILITY, STRENGTH, AND ENDURANCE

Athletes are always striving for ways to improve their performance and enhance their physical and mental wellbeing. Yoga can be an excellent tool for athletes to achieve these goals.

Flexibility is essential for athletes to perform at their best and avoid injury. Yoga poses can help increase flexibility by lengthening muscles and improving range of motion. For example, the seated forward bend can help increase hamstring flexibility, while the downward dog pose can stretch the calves, hamstrings, and spine.

Strength is also crucial for athletes—both in terms of performance and injury prevention. Practicing yoga can help strengthen muscles, especially when practicing challenging poses such as the plank or the warrior poses. These poses not only build muscle strength but also improve balance and stability.

Yoga can also help athletes enhance their endurance. The breathing techniques taught in yoga can improve lung capacity and help athletes sustain their physical activity for longer periods of time. Practicing yoga regularly can also help athletes become more aware of their body and its needs, allowing them to adjust their training and recovery strategies more effectively.

In addition to the physical benefits of yoga, it can also help athletes reduce stress and improve their mental wellbeing. Yoga requires a focused mind and can help improve concentration, which can be beneficial for athletes who need to maintain focus during competition. Practicing yoga can also help athletes cope with the stress of competition and improve their mental resilience.

Athletes who practice yoga can benefit in several ways, including increased flexibility, strength, endurance, and mental wellbeing. Incorporating yoga into a training routine can also help athletes avoid injury and promote recovery. Many professional athletes, from NBA players to Olympic gold medalists, have attested to the benefits of practicing yoga as a complement to their training regimen.

In conclusion, whether you are a professional athlete or a fitness enthusiast, practicing yoga can help you enhance your physical and mental wellbeing. Incorporating yoga into your training routine can improve your performance and reduce your risk of injury.

# PRENATAL YOGA: A SAFE AND EFFECTIVE WAY TO PREPARE FOR BIRTH

Pregnancy is one of the most beautiful experiences in life, and like most things in life, self-care is essential during this period. Prenatal yoga offers the ideal way to maintain physical and emotional health during pregnancy. Many expectant mothers experience a range of changes during pregnancy, such as back pain, fatigue, and insomnia. With prenatal yoga, you can alleviate these discomforts and expectations. This guide offers a complete guide to prenatal yoga, including its benefits and how to practice safely.

**The Benefits of Prenatal Yoga**

Prenatal yoga offers a range of benefits designed to promote the health of the mother and the baby. Some of the benefits include:

1. Increases flexibility: yoga helps to stretch the muscles, leading to improved flexibility and movement.

2. Reduces stress: prenatal yoga emphasizes relaxation techniques such as deep breathing and meditation, helping to reduce stress and create deep relaxation for the mother and baby.

3. Gives relief from back pain: during pregnancy, pressure builds up around the lower spine, leading to pain and discomfort. Prenatal yoga helps to stretch and strengthen the back muscles, reducing pain and discomfort.

4. Boosts energy: pregnant women often experience fatigue due to the demands of pregnancy. The breathing exercises, poses, and stretches offered in prenatal yoga help to improve energy levels,

helping the mother to cope with the physical and emotional changes experienced during pregnancy.

5. Improves sleep: prenatal yoga contributes to better sleep quality, helping the mother and baby to rest well and reduce the risk of complications from a lack of sleep.

## How to Practice Prenatal Yoga Safely

Before starting any form of exercise during pregnancy, you should consult your healthcare provider. Prenatal yoga poses are designed to be gentle, helping to avoid any strain that may lead to injury or affecting the baby. Here are a few tips on how to practice safely:

1. Find a certified prenatal yoga teacher: Yoga teachers with specialized training in prenatal yoga will be able to tailor the classes to your needs and provide safe modifications for any limitations or discomforts you may have.

2. Avoid twists and deep forward bends: These poses can create pressure on the stomach, increasing the risk of injury.

3. Use props: Blocks, blankets, and bolsters can offer support and ensure that you remain comfortable while sustaining poses.

4. Stay hydrated: Consume enough water to stay hydrated during these exercises to prevent dehydration and maintain a healthy pregnancy.

The above information provides a brief yet comprehensive guide to prenatal yoga. Always remember to listen to your body, practice safely, and consult your healthcare provider before starting prenatal yoga. With the right care, you can maintain physical, emotional, and mental health during your pregnancy while preparing for childbirth.

# SPECIAL CONSIDERATIONS FOR DIFFERENT BODY TYPES IN YOGA PRACTICE

Yoga is a practice that benefits everyone, regardless of body type, age, or physical ability. However, it's important to understand that there are different body types and what works for one may not work for another. It's necessary to consider individual differences during practice to avoid injury and maximize the benefits of yoga.

**Here are some special considerations to keep in mind for different body types when practicing yoga:**

For Petite Body Types
If you have a petite physique, it's important to focus on building strength and tone while maintaining flexibility. Try poses that promote muscle building, such as chair pose, warrior I and II, and downward-facing dog. These poses help increase core and arm strength while grounding through the legs.

For Plus Size Body Types
It's essential to focus on modifying poses and adapting practice to ensure safety and comfort when practicing yoga if you are plus-sized. Avoid putting pressure on joints and sensitive areas, such as the knees and lower back, and try out props such as chairs or straps to aid in practice. It's important to find modifications that work best for you and your body.

For Tall Body Types
Tall people should focus on poses that stretch the spine and help improve posture. Poses that promote proper alignment, such as mountain pose, standing forward bend, and downward-facing dog, help to stretch the legs and spine. Twists and inversions can

also be helpful for those with tall bodies.

For Short Limbs and Torso
People with short limbs and torso may need to modify their practice to accommodate their body type. It can be helpful to use props such as blocks or bolsters to help reach the ground during poses such as seated forward bends. Keep in mind poses that promote grounding can also help to create balance and stability.

For Curvy Body Types
Curvy people can benefit from practicing yoga in many ways, including building strength and increasing flexibility. Poses such as warrior I and II can help build strength while also improving posture. A well-rounded practice that incorporates both active and restorative poses can be helpful.

Regardless of your body type, it's important to listen to your body during practice and make modifications as needed. Finding a knowledgeable yoga teacher who is supportive and knowledgeable can help to tailor your practice to your body type and personal needs. Remember, yoga is all about finding inner peace, connecting with the breath, and finding balance, regardless of body type.

# YOGA PHILOSOPHY AND PRINCIPLES: THE DEEP ROOTS OF TRADITIONAL PRACTICE

Yoga is a practice that has been around for thousands of years and has evolved over time. While its benefits are widely recognized, not many people know the underlying philosophy and principles that make up the traditional practice of yoga. Understanding these principles can deepen your practice and help you integrate yoga into your daily life.

At the core of yoga philosophy are the concepts of self-realization and liberation. Yoga encourages individuals to look within themselves to find their true nature and to ultimately free themselves from suffering. This is achieved by following the eight limbs of yoga, which are outlined in Patanjali's Yoga Sutras, one of the foundational texts of yoga.

**The eight limbs of yoga include:**

1. Yama: ethical principles that guide our interactions with others, including nonviolence, truthfulness, non-stealing, moderation, and non-attachment.
2. Niyama: principles of personal discipline, including cleanliness, contentment, self-study, self-discipline, and surrender to a higher power.
3. Asana: physical postures meant to prepare the body for meditation and to increase physical health and strength.
4. Pranayama: breathing exercises designed to control the breath, increase energy, and calm the mind.
5. Pratyahara: withdrawal of the senses from external stimuli to focus inwardly.

6. Dharana: concentration, or the ability to hold the mind steady on a single point.
7. Dhyana: meditation, or the ability to maintain uninterrupted focus on an object.
8. Samadhi: a state of deep concentration where the individual experiences a sense of oneness with the universe.

Each limb builds upon the next, leading the individual towards self-realization and liberation. The physical postures or asanas that we commonly associate with yoga are just one small part of the practice. By incorporating all eight limbs of yoga, one can begin to transform body, mind, and spirit.

Additionally, the concept of ahimsa or non-violence is also a central principle in many of the modern branches of yoga. This means practicing kindness and compassion towards all living beings, including animals and the environment. By practicing non-violence towards yourself and others, you can cultivate a greater sense of peace and harmony in your life.

In summary, the philosophy and principles of yoga represent a holistic approach to self-improvement and well-being. Whether you are a beginner or an experienced practitioner, understanding the underlying principles of yoga can deepen your practice and help you live a more fulfilling life.

# YOGA AND AYURVEDA: INTEGRATING NUTRITION AND LIFESTYLE FOR MAXIMUM HEALTH BENEFITS

Ayurveda, a traditional Indian system of medicine, and yoga, a spiritual discipline that originated in ancient India, are two practices that complement each other in promoting overall health and well-being. Ayurveda focuses on balancing the body, mind, and spirit through lifestyle modifications, herbal remedies, and dietary changes, while yoga encompasses physical postures, breathing techniques, and meditation practices.

The principles of Ayurveda and yoga can be integrated to create a more comprehensive approach to health that addresses both the physical and the mental aspects of well-being. The combination of the two can help individuals achieve maximum health benefits.

Ayurveda emphasizes the importance of maintaining a balance between the three doshas: Vata, Pitta, and Kapha. Each individual has a unique combination of these doshas, and an imbalance can lead to various health problems. Similarly, yoga postures are designed to balance the body's energy centers or chakras, helping to restore the natural flow of energy throughout the body.

Diet plays a significant role in both Ayurveda and yoga, as food is considered a source of energy for the body. Ayurveda emphasizes the importance of eating fresh, whole foods that are rich in nutrients and avoiding processed, refined foods that are low in nutrition. Similarly, yoga practitioners emphasize the importance of a balanced diet that includes foods that provide energy and nourishment for the body.

Ayurveda prescribes specific diets based on an individual's doshas, and yoga practitioners recommend following a sattvic diet that includes fresh fruits, vegetables, whole grains, and legumes. Both Ayurveda and yoga place great emphasis on the digestive system, as good digestion is essential for good health.

Incorporating Ayurvedic practices into a yoga practice can enhance the overall healing benefits of yoga. For example, incorporating cleansing techniques known as kriyas in yoga practice can help remove toxins from the body, while Ayurvedic herbs can help boost immunity, improve digestion, and promote relaxation.

In conclusion, combining Ayurveda and yoga offers a holistic approach to health and wellness that addresses the body, mind, and spirit. Integrating Ayurvedic principles into a yoga practice can enhance the overall benefits, promoting overall health and well-being.

# YOGA AND MINDFULNESS: A HOLISTIC APPROACH TO WELLNESS

More and more people are turning to mindfulness and yoga as holistic approaches to wellness. While both practices have unique benefits individually, combining them can lead to a more profound experience in healing the mind and body.

Mindfulness is the practice of being present in the moment, observing your thoughts and feelings without judgment. It's a powerful tool that can help you manage stress, improve focus and concentration, and cultivate a deeper sense of peace and contentment. Yoga, on the other hand, is an ancient practice that combines physical postures (asanas), breathing techniques (pranayama), and meditation to promote physical, mental, and emotional well-being.

When practiced together, the benefits of both mindfulness and yoga are amplified. During a yoga session, practicing mindfulness can help you deepen your poses and improve your own reaction to negative thoughts in your mind. While on the other hand, yoga can help you release stored tension and stress in your body, making it easier to relax into a state of mindfulness.

There are different ways to integrate mindfulness and yoga into your daily routine, and here are some ideas on how to get started:

1. Meditate Before Starting Your Yoga Practice: Start by setting aside a few minutes to clear your mind through meditation. With a few deep breaths and focused attention, you can ground yourself in the present moment, and prepare your mind and body for your yoga practice.

2. Practice Mindful Breathing: During your yoga practice, pay close attention to your breath. Breathe fully and deeply, inhaling and exhaling mindfully, and cultivate focus on the way your breath flows in and out of your body.

3. Incorporate Mindfulness during the Entire Yoga Sequence: Whenever your mind wanders, try to bring it back to the sensations in your body, the rhythm of your breath, and the present moment. This will increase the effectiveness of yoga to reach deeper states of relaxation and improve your overall wellness.

4. Take Mindful Moments off the Mat: Practice mindful moments off the mat during your daily routine—whether it's taking a deep breath before eating, or taking mindful steps during a walk, practicing mindfulness even for many small moments each day can lead to significant benefits.

Yoga and mindfulness are complementary practices that support each other in promoting holistic well-being. Incorporating both into your daily routine can make a huge difference in your mental, physical and emotional health.

# CHOOSING A YOGA TEACHER AND PRACTICING SAFELY: TIPS FOR BEGINNERS AND ADVANCED YOGIS.

Yoga is a great way to improve your physical and mental health. However, it's important to practice it safely and under the guidance of a qualified teacher. Choosing the right yoga teacher and practicing safely can ensure you get the most out of your yoga practice and avoid injury. Here are some tips for beginners and advanced yogis.

1. Research Before You Choose: There are different types of yoga and styles, and each instructor has a unique teaching approach. Do some research to find a teacher who matches your requirements. You can check websites, social media platforms, or reviews from friends and relatives who practice yoga.

2. Check Certifications of the Teacher: Ensure the yoga teacher has completed a certification program recognized by Yoga Alliance as they set minimum requirements for yoga teacher training. Moreover, look out for yoga studios, which are also registered with Yoga Alliance as they ensure studio safety and standardized yoga classes.

3. Observe a Class: Before committing to a class, it is important to attend a few trial sessions. It enables you to observe the instructor, class, and the studio. It is the best way to assess their teaching style, the difficulty level of the class, and the group dynamic.

4. Inform the Instructor about Your Medical History: It's essential to inform the instructor of any injuries or medical conditions

so that they can adapt poses accordingly. Any medical history, including past surgeries or illnesses, should be shared to avoid any complications.

5. Listen to Your Body and Take Breaks as Needed: Do not push beyond your physical capacity. Listen to your body, take breaks if required, and never compare yourself to others. Yoga is not a competition, and you do not have to go beyond your limits to prove your capability.

6. Use Props: Yoga props such as blocks or straps help beginners and advanced yogis to get into proper alignment more easily or can adjust poses to fit their needs. Don't hesitate to use them, even the most experienced yogis use props when necessary.

7. Be Patient: Developing a consistent yoga practice requires patience, and it takes time to see results. It's important not to get discouraged and keep practicing regularly. You will see improvements slowly over time.

In conclusion, choosing a yoga teacher and practicing safely should not be taken lightly. By taking the time to research, observe classes, and communicate your health status with your yoga teacher, you can enjoy the numerous benefits that yoga offers. Remember, yoga is not just about flexibility or strength, it's a wholesome approach to living a healthier and happier life.